Yoga For Fat Guys

The Short Attention Span Guide:

Yoga For Fat Guys

FROM LUMPY TO LIMBER IN JUST WEEKS

John J. Gillies,
Artwork by Jill Krynicki
Foreword by Dr. Michael T. Wayda, D.C.

Sawle Register Service
Madison

The information this book reflects the opinion of the author. In no way is it to be considered medical advice. Specific medical advice should be obtained from a licensed medical professional. You should consult with your health care provider before beginning this program, any other health improvement regimen or lifestyle change. This information is in no way meant to treat, cure or prevent any disease or illness from happening.

First published 2009 in the United States by Sawle Register Service.

All illustrations by Jill Krynicki

ISBN: 978-0-9824750-0-3

To my family and friends.

Foreword

When I was asked to read, <u>Short-Attention Span Guide: Yoga for Fat Guys</u>, I was pleasantly surprised by the simplicity in the instructions and the diagrams. Finally; a book that could help make Yoga more accessible to the people that need it the most; and that includes me. I was especially impressed with the warm-up and other tips found throughout the book.

My name is Dr. Michael Wayda. John and I met when he came to me after suffering neck and upper back injuries in a car accident. His injuries were severe and included "Whiplash" and a concussion. The pain and muscle spasms caused by these injuries left John immobilized.

Chiropractic adjustments, physiotherapy and rehabilitative exercises helped John to heal quickly from his extensive injuries. John proved to be an excellent patient because he was more in tune with his body than most, if not all, of my other patients. John followed instructions and challenged me to help him recover as fast as possible.

I see that John has collected many of his past experiences and infused them into the text and his animator did a wonderful job of showing the exercises in his book <u>Yoga for Fat Guys</u>. Overall; I highly recommend that anyone buy this book and start living a more healthy and enjoyable life.

<u>Yoga for Fat Guys</u> was born from one man's journey to find health and wellness. I hope you all have as much fun with this book as I have enjoyed.

Dr. Michael Wayda

Author's Notes

I'm an expert at being overweight. I've struggled with my weight almost all of my adult life. On two different occasions, I have ballooned up to almost 300 pounds. I'm only 6 feet tall, so it's hard to hide the fact that I'm carrying so much extra weight. Many of you will complain that I cannot be an expert. You will say that I am not a doctor, nutritionist or other medical professional. You are correct. I did not say I am an expert on the physiological effects of being overweight.

I am an expert on *actually being overweight*. On the enormous physical and mental toll it has taken on me over the past 30 years.

Yoga for Fat Guys is not a be-all and end-all yoga book. If the author of a book about yoga declares: "This is the authoritative yoga book! All other yoga books are wrong and false!", then they are lying to you. Yoga is a huge topic. This book presents a very small slice of yoga that I modified to meet my needs. I firmly believe that my method will meet the needs of many other fat people.

A few notes regarding the text. I'm a man and I wrote this book for other men, therefore I use male pronouns throughout the book. There may be a time and a place for political correctness, but it's not here. This book is written to provide guidance for fat people who want to improve their lives. Some people may be offended by some of the things that are written in this book. I have chosen the risk of offending some to provide greater benefit to others.

Thanks,
John Gillies
Summer, 2009

Contents

The Basics

The Exercises

The Yoga Poses

Making It Work

Weight Loss

Appendix

Introduction

The reason you don't do yoga is psychological. You have a mental block. You don't do yoga because you don't think you can do yoga. Yoga intimidates you. Yoga intimidates you because it appears to be practiced by a small group of perfect physical specimens happily moving from pose to pose without a care in the world. It intimidates you when you walk past the yoga books in the bookstore or the library.

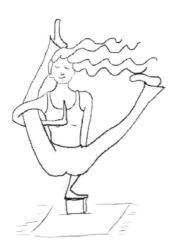

Right there on the cover is some perfect little woman with perfect little boots and a perfect little butt and a perfect little smile. In many cases, she is twisted into a yoga pose that not even Gumby can do. Yoga intimidates you when you see it on TV. You're sitting on the couch, happily channel surfing and waiting for the pizza man to arrive. Suddenly, "happy pretzel woman" has invaded your space and is right there on your TV.

It's easy to see why this intimidates you. The woman on the book cover is in tremendous physical shape, while you are woefully out of shape. Most people subconsciously place a high value on physical fitness. This is probably true for you as well. You are making a value judgment and comparing yourself to "happy pretzel woman". You cannot possibly compete with her, so you decide that you are unable to do yoga before you even try it.

It's not that you don't want to be in shape and flexible. You've probably said (or thought) something like: "I wish I could do that!" You know that being flexible and in shape are good things. The problem is you do not know if you can pay the price to get back in shape. You look at "happy pretzel woman", and then you look at yourself and it just seems hopeless. The result is that you surrender before you start.

This book was written to level the playing field. "Happy pretzel woman" has probably been doing yoga for years, maybe even decades. She can get into those poses because she has years of practice. It's possible that she has been

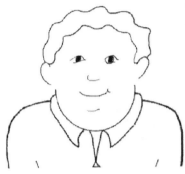

doing yoga since before you were born. Comparing yourself to her is unfair. You need to compare yourself to someone who is fat and out of shape.

Meet Burl. Burl is the star of Yoga for Fat Guys.

Burl is one of us. He is overweight, but he used to be in pretty good shape. He leads a sedentary life, but he used to be very active. He works in the cubicle farm 40 hours a week, struggling to make ends meet. His schedule prevents him from playing the team sports he enjoys. His shirts are all too tight, he has trouble bending over and he feels stiff and sore all the time.

He has tried fad diets, exercise machines, health clubs and miracle products advertised on infomercials. Everything has kind of worked for a little while, but in the end it has all fallen flat. The reason none of these things worked is because Burl did not have the time and energy to invest in them. He needs something that does not require a lot of time, can be done without any special equipment and is easy to remember. He also wants something that is inexpensive and does not have a bunch of fine print.

Yoga for Fat Guys worked for Burl. Give it the chance to work for you.

The Basics

Warming Up

Most books about exercise have extensive sections on warming up. Warming up is very important, but it's only a part of the exercise routine. The warm-up should not take longer than the work out.

It's going to take you longer to warm up than a skinny person simply because you're fat. Logically, the more overweight you are the more you're going to have to do to get properly loosened up.

A simple way to warm up quickly is to walk in place lifting your knees as high as you can and clenching and unclenching your fists in rhythm. Count to yourself while you are walking in place. Your count is "one-two-three-one", "one-two-three-two" up to "one-two-three-sixty". This should take you one or two minutes. This warm-up should be adequate for most of you.

Here's another warm-up you can do if you feel you are still not quite loose enough: Turn on your radio or MP3 player and find a song that you like. The songs have kind of a quick tempo and last about three minutes. Simply dance in place for the duration of this song. Don't go wild and berserk while dancing-a variant of "The Twist" works just fine. When you are done dancing in place, you should be properly warmed up.

Some of you may be very stiff. Now we have what's known as a "Catch-22": you need to loosen up because you're fat but you can't loosen up because you're fat. You probably need some help getting loose. You may even need to use tools to get loose. In those cases, take a hot shower. Take a four to five minute shower that is as hot as you can tolerate. The reason for this is simple: the heat of the shower combined with the beat of the water against your body will get your blood moving.

When you leave the shower, dry yourself off quickly and begin walking and dancing in place.

Determining Your Baseline

Your baseline is nothing more than your starting point. It's where you are today and it's influenced by a many different factors. These factors include, but are not limited to, height, weight, age, percent body fat, normal level of physical activity, diet, stress, etc. Changes in the baseline over time are how you will measure your progress.

To measure your baseline you will need a chair, a timer and a pen or pencil.

The procedure for measuring your baseline is very simple. You will begin the procedure seated in a chair:

1. Start the timer.

2. Assume the "Power" pose.

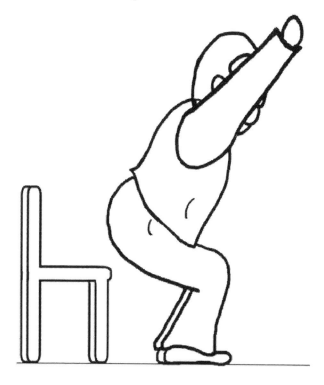

3. Hold the pose until you are physically unable to maintain it.

4. Write down how long you were able to maintain the pose (measure the time to the nearest second).

5. Rest for two minutes.

6. Repeat steps one through five.

7. Repeat steps one through five again.

8. Find the total number of seconds you were in the "Power" pose.

This total is your baseline. You should check your baseline at least once a month.

On days when you check your baseline, it should always be the first thing you do in your workout. You should do the baseline check immediately after your warm up.

.

The Exercises

The Asana (The Prayer Pose)

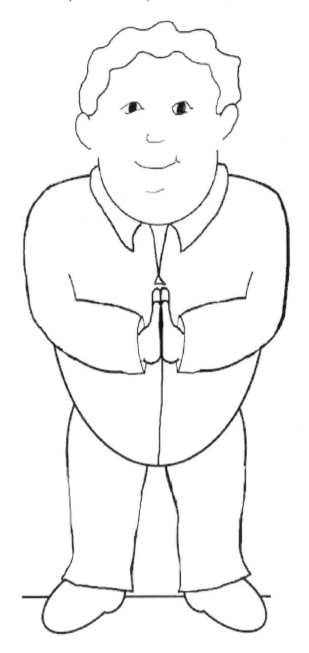

Type: Isometric.

Develops: Upper body strength and endurance.

Position: Standing with feet normal width apart.

Alternate Position: Seated with feet on the floor normal width apart and back straight.

Description: Put your hands together, palms facing inward. The fingers and thumbs should be touching each other and your thumbs should be touching your chest. Your forearms should be parallel to the ground.

Exercise: Push your hands together as hard as you are able. Keep your head, neck, lower back and legs relaxed. Exert even pressure until you begin to feel discomfort in your arms or you begin to breathe hard. Maintain the exercise for about 15 seconds after you feel discomfort or notice that you are breathing hard.

Notes: This position is based upon a traditional Hindu greeting. Trekkers may also recognize this as a traditional Vulcan greeting.

Atlas (The Beer Vendor Pose)

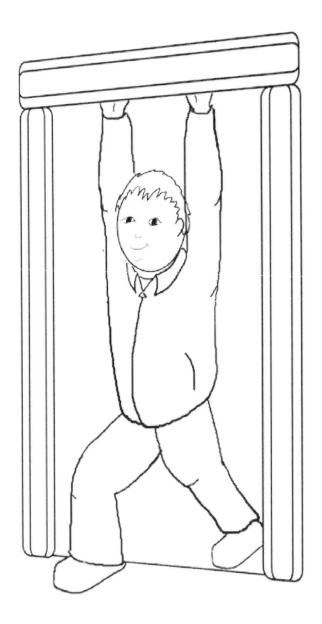

Type: Isometric.

Develops: Overall strength and endurance.

Position: Standing under a doorway with the front foot extended.

Alternate Position: None.

Description: Place the palms of your hands on the top of the doorframe. Extend your arms and lock your elbows. Keep your back straight; relax your head and neck. The feet are normal width apart. Extend one foot forward while keeping both heels firmly on the ground.

Exercise: Press vertically against the door frame with all your might. Keep your head and neck relaxed. Exert steady pressure until you begin to begin to breathe hard or feel discomfort in your arms, legs or back. Maintain the exercise for about 15 seconds after you notice that you are breathing hard or feeling discomfort in your arms legs or back.

Notes: This exercise is based on the mythical figure Atlas. You can also picture this exercise as a beer vendor carrying a case of beer through the bleachers at Wrigley Field.

Bridge

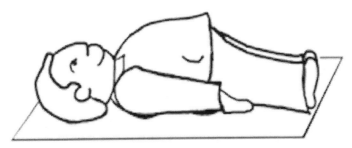

Bridge position 1: Lay on your back and relax.

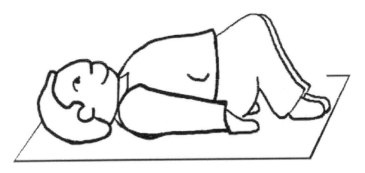

Bridge position 2: Bring your heels as close to
your butt as you can.

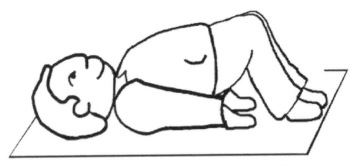

Bridge position 3: Slowly raise your butt off the
floor without lifting your shoulder blades

Type: Isometric.

Develops: Abdominal strength, leg strength and endurance.

Position: Lay flat on your back on a firm surface. Do not use your bed or a couch. The knees are bent and the soles of the feet rest flat on the ground. Your arms are relaxed at your sides and your head and neck are relaxed. You should use a mat if you have one.

Alternate Position: None.

Description: Your lower back, buttocks and legs are raised, forming a small arch.

Exercise: Flex your buttocks while slowly raising your pelvis off the floor. It should feel like the bones of your spine are coming up off the floor one after another. You should stop raising your pelvis when you feel your shoulder blade began to lift. If you raise your shoulder blades off the floor, you'll put too much stress on your neck. Maintain that position until you feel discomfort in your abdomen or legs or until you begin to breathe hard. Maintain the exercise for about 15 seconds after you notice the discomfort or that you are breathing hard.

If your legs cramp during this exercise, stop immediately.

Notes: This exercise is a variant of a wrestling drill known as "bridging".

You can help keep your upper spine properly aligned by placing a rolled up towel under your neck during this exercise.

If you cramp up during this exercise, walk it off and refer to the section on cramping at the end of the book.

Plank

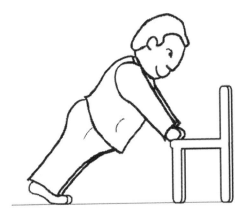

Beginning Plank Position: Use a chair
to keep your hands above your feet.

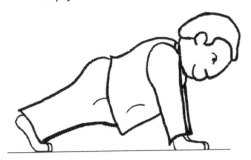

Intermediate Plank Position: Keep your body
straight and lock your elbows.

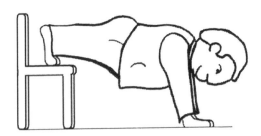

Advanced Plank Position: Use a chair
to keep your feet above your head.

Type: Isometric.

Develops: Overall body strength and endurance.

Position: The up position of the push-up.

Alternate Position: None.

Description: The "up position" of the push-up (many of you may consider this position mythical or legendary).

Exercise: Hold the position until you begin to breathe hard or you experience discomfort in your arms, then hold the position for about 15 more seconds.

If your arms cramp up during this exercise, stop immediately.

Notes: This exercise can be made more challenging by placing the feet on an object so that the feet are above the hands.

Work hard to keep your spine properly aligned during this exercise.

If you cramp up during this exercise, walk it off and refer to the section on cramping at the end of the book.

Power

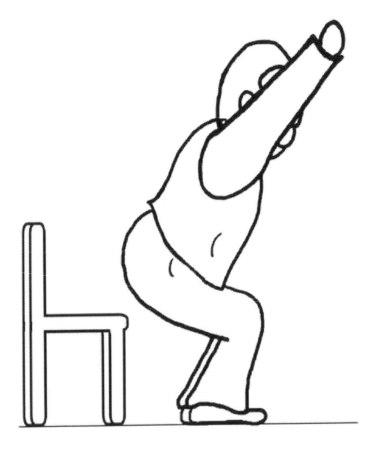

The Power Position: Always start and end this pose seated comfortably in a sturdy chair near a sturdy desk or table.

Type: Isometric.

Develops: Lower body strength and endurance.

Position: Sit in a chair with your arms and hands extended over your head. Clench your fists and lock your elbows. Look straight ahead, relax your neck and keep your back straight.

Alternate Position: Clasp your hands together above your head.

Description: A modified sitting position.

Exercise: Lift your buttocks about three inches off of the chair. Hold this position until you begin breathing hard or began to feel discomfort in your legs. Then hold the position for 15 more seconds.

Stop the exercise and sit down immediately if your legs cramp up, you lose your balance or otherwise feel this position has become unsafe.

Notes: This exercise is also used for self evaluation purposes.

Work hard to keep your spine properly aligned during this exercise.

If you cramp up during this exercise, walk it off and refer to the section on cramping at the end of the book.

Samson

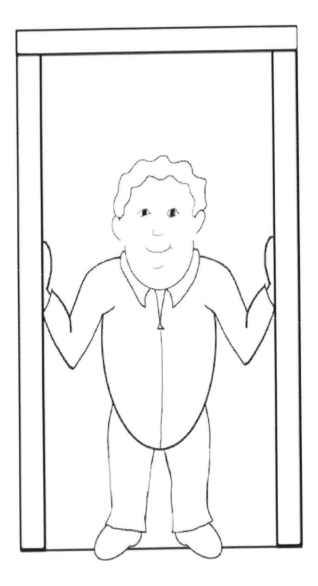

This pose can be done between any two solid objects.

Type: Isometric.

Develops: Upper body strength and endurance.

Position: Stand in a doorway with your feet normal width apart.

Alternate Position: None.

Description: Stand in a doorway and extend your arms. Grasp the door frame at about shoulder height. Look straight ahead and relax your head and neck.

Exercise: Press outward with all of your might against the door frame until you feel discomfort in your arms or you begin to breathe hard. Then hold the pose for about 15 more seconds.

Notes: This pose is named after the biblical hero Samson.

Toe Lifts

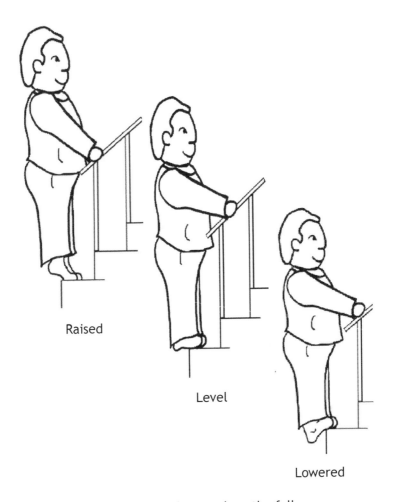

Raised

Level

Lowered

These three figures show the full
range of motion for toe lifts.

Type: Isotonic.

Develops: Lower leg strength, endurance and balance.

Position: Stand with your knees locked and your feet normal width apart. Place your toes on the edge of a stair with your heels hanging over the edge. Keep your head and neck relaxed while looking straight ahead.

Alternate Position: You can use any elevated step. Many vehicles have excellent platforms for this exercise as well. Some examples include the tailgate of a golf cart, the side doors of most minivans and the running boards of many medium duty trucks.

Alternate Method: You can do this exercise one leg at a time. Just let your other leg "hang" in the air.

Description: A modified standing position.

Exercise: Raise or lower your feet to a predetermined position and hold that position until you breathe hard. Then relax for 15 seconds and repeat three times.

Alternate Exercise: Raise and lower your body using only your toes. Move smoothly and evenly through your full range of motion several times until you get tired, then continue for about fifteen more seconds.

Notes: You can even do this exercise while waiting for the bus. Simply let your heels hang over the edge of the curb and use the bus stop sign for balance. If anybody asks what you are doing, you can tell them you are superhero preparing for a day of fighting villainy. It's (probably) not true, but it's fun to see how people react.

X Factor Arms (Wolverine)

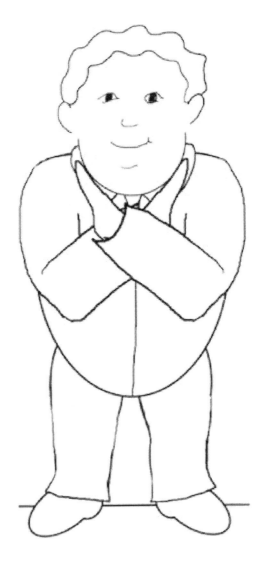

Wolverine (Titanium claws not shown).

Type: Isometric.

Develops: Upper body strength and endurance.

Position: Stand with your feet normal width apart. Look forward while relaxing your head and neck. Cross your arms in front of your chin with the forearms touching.

Alternate Position: You can do this exercise sitting down or laying on a mat.

Description: A modified standing position.

Exercise: Press your forearms together with all your might. Hold this position for about 15 seconds after you begin breathing hard. Relax for one minute, reverse the position of your arms and repeat.

Notes: Feel free to tape kitchen knives to your knuckles during this exercise. You will look and *feel* just like Wolverine™.†

†: I know a good gag when I steal it and I stole the Wolverine™ gag from *8 Simple Rules for Buying My Teenage Daughter*, an episode of the fourth season of Family Guy.

X Factor Legs

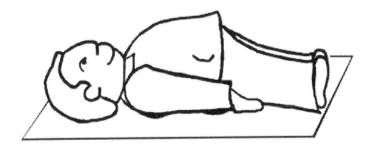

X-Factor Legs: Up position. Relax your body and place
a rolled-up towel under your neck.

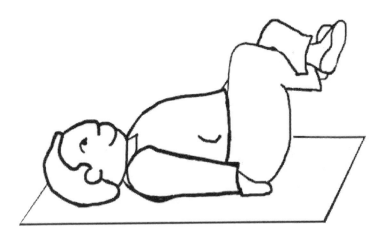

X-Factor Legs: Up position. Keep your upper-body
relaxed during the exercise.

Type: Isometric.

Develops: Lower body strength and endurance.

Position: Lay down on a smooth, firm surface. Support your neck with a towel. Your head and neck are relaxed. Rest your arms in any comfortable position. Bring your knees up to your chest and cross your lower legs above the ankle.

Alternate Position: None.

Description: See start position.

Exercise: Press your legs together with all your might. Hold this position for about 15 seconds after you begin breathing hard. Relax for one minute, reverse the position of your legs and repeat.

Notes: If possible, keep your entire upper body relaxed during this exercise.

The Yoga Poses

Downward Facing Dog

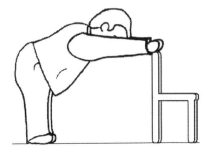

Beginners should use
A sturdy high-backed
chair as a brace for
their first few
sessions.

Intermediate users should
spin the chair around and
use the seat of the chair
as a brace while their
flexibility improves.

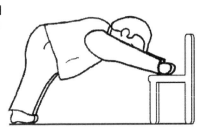

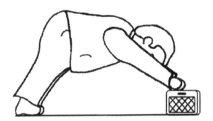

Advanced users can
replace the chair
with a sturdy solid
object like a milk
crate.

Expert users should
place their hands
directly on the floor.
Eventually, you will be
able to place the palms
of your hands next to
your feet.

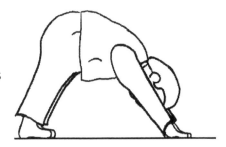

Type: Traditional

Develops: Flexibility and endurance.

Start Position: Stand with your feet normal width apart. Relax your head and neck and look straight ahead.

Alternate Start Positions: Plank, Upward Facing Dog or on your hands and knees.

Description: Your body bends at the waist to form an inverted "V" shape.

Posing: While standing, extend your hands over your head. Lean forward from your ankles and bend at the waist. Keep your heels on the ground throughout the exercise. Continue bending forward until you can place the palms of your hands on the floor. Keep your back and legs as straight as possible. If you are a beginner or an intermediate user, place your hands on a raised surface like a table, chair or milk crate. Hold this pose until you begin to breathe hard.

Notes: If possible, keep your entire upper body relaxed during this exercise.

Tree

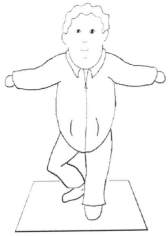

Tree Pose for beginners. Work at developing your balance. Touch your heel to your calf and extend your arms at shoulder height.

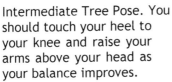

Intermediate Tree Pose. You should touch your heel to your knee and raise your arms above your head as your balance improves.

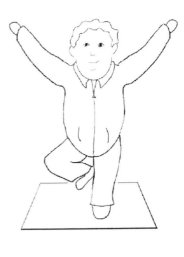

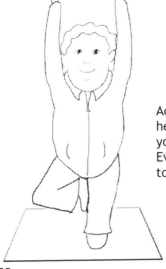

Advanced Tree Pose. Touch your heel to your thigh and extend your arms above your head. Eventually, you will be able to touch your heel to your butt.

Type: Traditional

Develops: Balance and endurance.

Start Position: Stand with your feet normal width apart. Relax your whole body and look straight ahead.

Alternate Start Positions: None.

Description: Stand on one leg while posing with your arms and your other leg.

Posing: Place the sole of your raised foot against to the inside of your base leg. Over time, you will be able to raise your foot higher as your balance and flexibility improve. Eventually, your raised foot will be touching your butt. Your arm movements should be even and steady throughout the exercise.

Notes: Many of you have lost a great deal of your coordination and your sense of balance. This is normal for people who lead sedentary lifestyles. This loss is not permanent, and your balance will improve over time if you do the exercises. This means is that you may have to use the beginner or intermediate poses of this exercise for a while.

Triangle

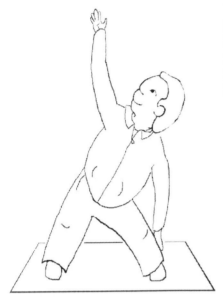

The Triangle Poses:
Start Position.
Place your hand on
your knee, extend
your other hand above
your head and stretch.

←

The Triangle Poses:
End Position.
Your lower hand has
slid further down your
leg and your other
arm is fully extended.

After a few sessions,
your hand will touch
your foot and after a
few more sessions,
you will be able to
place your palm on
the floor.

→

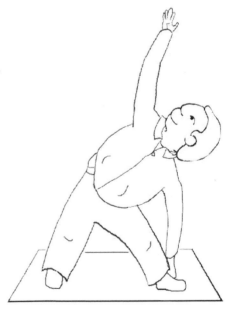

Type: Traditional

Develops: Lateral stability and endurance.

Start Position: Stand with your feet wider than normal, relax your whole body and look straight ahead.

Alternate Start Positions: None.

Description: Form a triangle with your torso, one of your legs and one of your arms. Extend your other arm straight up into the air. Keep both of your heels on the ground and look at your raised hand.

Posing: DO NOT BOUNCE OR JERK INTO POSITION. Slide one hand as far down your leg as possible. Do not lean forward. After sliding your hand as far down your side as possible, extend your other hand upward. Your gaze follows this hand as it reaches upward. Stretch as far as you can and then hold for about fifteen seconds.

After resting for about one minute, repeat the pose with the arms reversed.

Notes: DO NOT BOUNCE OR JERK INTO POSITION. This pose is all about being smooth. Your massive gut leads to an increased chance of pulling or tearing one of your Intercostal muscles if you bounce or jerk during this exercise. Your range of motion will probably be quite limited the first few times you do this pose. That's OK. The goal of this exercise is to enhance your mobility. Eventually, you will be able to widen your stance beyond the diagrams shown in this book and your hand will touch your ankle with ease.

Upward Facing Dog

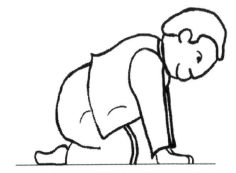

Start the Upward Facing Dog on all fours.

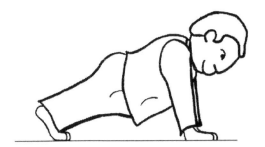

Extend your feet to the rear to
assume the Plank position.

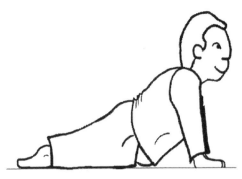

Roll your toes to the rear, thrust your chest forward,
press your hips down and arch your neck.

Type: Traditional

Develops: Flexibility in the torso.

Start Position: On your hands and knees.

Alternate Start Positions: You can start from either the Plank position or the Upward Facing Dog.

Description: Like a wolf howling at the moon.

Posing: Extend your toes as far to the rear as possible with the tops of your feet touching the floor. Lock your elbows, push your abdomen toward the floor, arch your back, thrust your chest forward and point your chin and look upward as far as you can. Hold the pose for about 15 seconds after you begin breathing hard.

Notes: Advanced users should move between Upward Facing Dog and Downward Facing Dog two or three times in succession.

Warrior

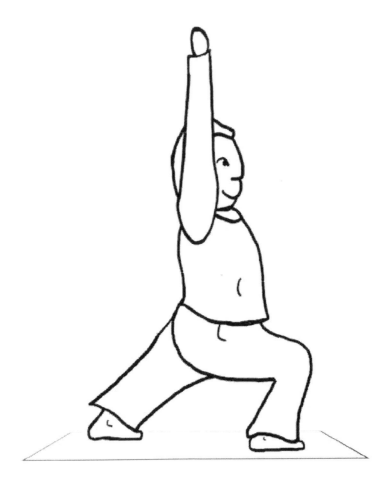

The Warrior Pose with the arms extended overhead. Keep both heels on the ground while moving your arms through the full range of motion and rotating your torso at the waist.

Type: Traditional

Develops: Flexibility in the torso and endurance.

Start Position: stand with one foot forward or extended, relax and look straight ahead.

Alternate Start Positions: None.

Description: A variation of the Atlas exercise.

Posing: Press your front knee forward and keep both heels on the ground. Thrust your chest forward, arch your back and tuck your chin. Extend your arms to the sides, parallel to the ground with the palms up.

Slowly bring your hands together above your head, and then lower them again.

Keep moving your arms through this range of motion until you begin to breathe hard or your arms or legs cramp up.

Notes: You can rotate your torso at the waist for variety.

Half Moon

Type: Traditional

Develops: Comprehensive exercise.

Start Position: Tree (intermediate position).

Alternate Start Positions: None.

Description: At the end of the sequence, your pose will resemble a half moon. This is the only really "advanced" pose included in <u>Yoga for Fat Guys</u>. It is also the only pose that requires several position changes, works your whole body and takes a long time to develop.

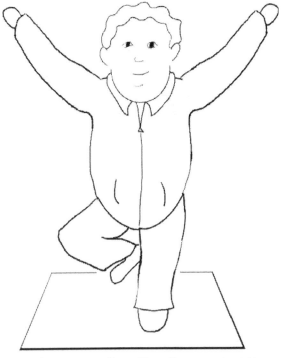

Use the Intermediate Tree Pose to start the
Half Moon Pose

Half Moon (continued)

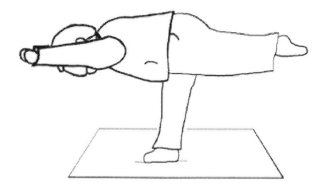

Extend your raised leg behind you and extend your hands above your head. Flex at the waist so your torso and raised leg are parallel to the ground.

This position is known as "The Spearman" and it is an excellent tool if you are having balance issues.

Half Moon (continued)

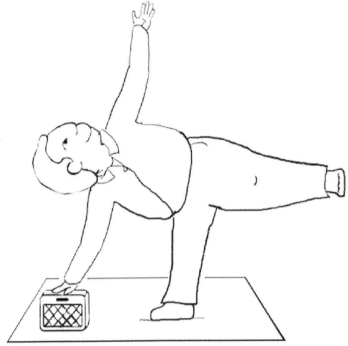

Rotate your torso and extend your arms. Place your lower
hand on a solid object like a milk crate, foot stool or
cinder block.

This pose is called **The Supported Half Moon**.

Half Moon (continued)

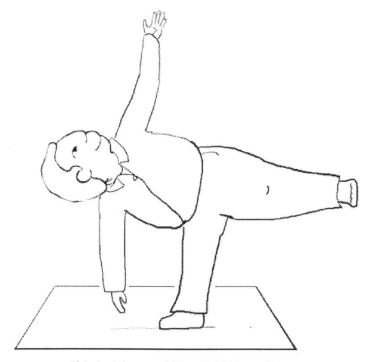

This is **Advanced The Half Moon Pose.**

Remove your hand from the support. You should have one
available, but only use it to regain your balance.
Your goal should be to hold this pose for one minute
without using a support.

Change legs and repeat: Your legs are not exactly alike and
one of your legs will be better at this pose than the other.
This is normal and it is because one of your legs is stronger
and more stable than the other leg. Additionally, your sense
of balance changes as your position changes. Change your
legs and repeat the Half Moon Pose to develop strength in
your other leg and improve your overall sense of balance.

Making it Work

Do <u>Yoga for Fat Guys</u> on a regular basis

Ideally, you should do <u>Yoga for Fat Guys</u> two days in a row, then take one day off. Develop a regular schedule and stick to it.

Rest between Exercises

When you begin doing <u>Yoga for Fat Guys</u>, rest for three minutes between exercises. Reduce your rest interval to two minutes after the first month and then reduce it one minute after the third month.

Dealing with Fatigue and Exhaustion

These exercises are intense, especially if you are obese or have lived a sedentary lifestyle for a long time. You will reach a point where you are fatigued. That's OK. Increase your rest interval and continue. If you are still fatigued, shorten the time you spend doing each exercise or holding each pose.

It's important that you attempt each pose, even if your attempt is only for a few seconds. Don't get discouraged and quit. Hang tough because the results are worth the effort.

Cramping

Cramps should be massaged out quickly to prevent more serious injuries.

Leg Cramps: These are the most common cramps and the easiest to manage. Walk until the cramp stops, then massage the area and apply warm moist towels to relax the muscles.

Other Cramps: Proceed directly to massage and moist heat.

Frequent Cramps: If you develop cramps every time you exercise, you may need vitamins or minerals. Contact your health care provider and get advice specific to your situation.

Temporary Relief: Calcium based antacid tablets like Tums can be used for temporary relief from cramps.

Additional Physical Activity

Yoga for Fat Guys is a good start, but you should add some other physical activities to your life. Here are some examples:

- If you have an active sex life, have more sex.

- Shoot baskets a few times a week.

- Play "catch" with a wall. Pick up a tennis ball and an old baseball glove.

- Hit a bucket at the driving range.

- Take the stairs.

- Park your car two or three blocks from work and walk the rest of the way.

- Use the stairs.

  The list is endless.

  Participants in every sport have developed cheap methods to practice and prepare for the sport. Many of these methods provide a good workout, are easily portable and can often be purchased for pennies on the dollar at garage sales, used sporting goods stores or online.

If you are able, you should add about 30 minutes of aerobics to your routine two or three times a week. There is an excellent collection of classic videos available for free online at www.jacklalanne.com . Mr. LaLanne is an American icon. He is the granddaddy of them all. He was the first person to bring exercise, health and fitness to the masses through television. A collection of his TV shows is available for free at his website. The music may be dated and the graphics are primitive, but he provides exercises and advice in those videos that stand the test of time. These videos are a valuable tool and are definitely worth watching.

44

Weight Loss

There is no mystery to weight loss. If you spend more calories than you eat, you will lose weight.

You may need some background information in order to understand how people gain and lose weight.

A calorie is a unit of energy. A dietary calorie is simply 1000 calories. A pound of fat contains approximately 3500 dietary calories.

This means that you will gain 1 pound of fat for every 3500 excess calories that you eat. On the other hand, you will lose 1 pound of fat if you spend 3500 more calories than you eat. The effect is cumulative and it is not time sensitive. There is no "expiration date" on weight gain or weight loss. If you consume 3500 excess calories in one week, you will gain 1 pound of fat at the end of that week. If you expend 3500 calories more than you consume over the course of one week, then you will lose 1 pound of fat. This is true if the timeframe is weeks or months or years.

A Three Part Plan For Weight Loss

There are three parts to any successful weight loss plan:

1. Increase the calories you expend

2. Decrease the calories you consume

3. Monitor your progress

Increase The Calories You Expend

Increasing the calories you expend means being more active. The following examples assume you weigh 275 pounds and that you exert a reasonable effort. The actual number of calories you spend will depend on how much you weigh and how hard you work.

- If you do 30 minutes of <u>Yoga for Fat Guys</u> five times a week, then you will burn and additional 900 calories per week.

- If you add 20 minutes of brisk walking 3 days a week, you will burn an additional 450 calories each week.

- If you shoot baskets for 20 minutes three times per week, you will burn an additional 550 calories each week.

Adding these three activities to your weekly routine will burn an additional 1900 calories per week

Decrease The Calories You Consume

You need to have an effective the eating plan if you are going to lose weight and keep it off. Start by compiling a journal of what you eat, and then look for ways to save calories by substitution or portion reduction.

- A typical doughnut contains 300 calories, but a granola bar only has 120 calories. Many fat people routinely eat two doughnuts every day during breakfast. If you make this switch you will "save" 360 calories a day. You will cut 1800 calories each week if you make this switch Monday through Friday.

- Change your snacking habits. A candy bar from the vending machine has about 150 calories, but a piece of string cheeses contains only about 50 calories. You will cut 500 calories if you replace one chocolate bar a day with a piece of string cheese five times per week.

- You can save a ton of calories by replacing potato chips with fresh fruit. If you have a large grapefruit instead of a bag of chips from a vending machine you will cut about 175 calories. If you make this replacement five times a week, you cut almost 900 calories each week.

Making these dietary changes will cut your caloric intake 3200 calories every week.

Monitor Your Progress

Your bathroom scale will be a source of constant temptation and frustration. Every day you will step on the scale, expecting huge weight losses. Every day you will get depressed because weight loss is a process that takes time. There is only one way to handle this situation.

Throw away your bathroom scale!

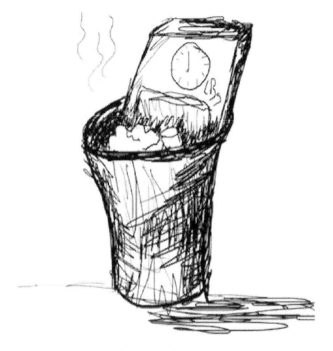

There are three methods to monitor your progress.

1. The Lazy method

2. The "Button-Down Shirt" method

3. The "Anal Retentive" method

The Lazy Method

Get a simple heath screening. Have the provider check your weight, blood pressure and heart rate. Do this every six months and keep track of the results.

The "Button-Down Shirt" Method

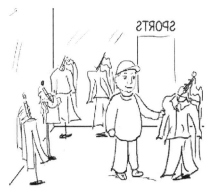

Purchase a shirt that is one size too small for you. Try it on once a week. Eventually, you will be able to button all the buttons and move around without popping a button or bursting a seam. At this point, buy yourself a few new shirts as a reward. You should also purchase another shirt that is one size too small and repeat the process.

The "Anal Retentive" Method

Keep a daily journal of your activities and emotions. Write down the activities that are more difficult because you are fat. Write down the emotional stresses and strains caused by your extra weight. Analyze what's happening to you over time. Look for areas that have improved and identify areas that need improvement.

Exercise versus Diet

The exercise program in <u>Yoga for Fat Guys</u> is geared to improving your strength, endurance and flexibility, but it will help you lose weight. You will need to invest six hours each week in the exercise program. You will burn 1900 additional calories per week on this program.

Controlling your diet is far more important to managing your weight than exercise. Controlling your diet is also easier to do, takes less time and costs less money than exercise does. In the example above, three simple dietary substitutions reduced caloric intake by 3200 calories per week.

- Dietary substitutions are easy; all you have to do is go to a different aisle in the grocery store. Exercise is hard because you have to actually do the exercise.

- Dietary substitutions take no time at all, but you have to set time aside to exercise.

- You might actually *save money* by making dietary substitutions, but you might need to spend a few bucks on exercise gear.

This comparison may seem to say "Don't exercise, just diet". I encourage you not to follow that path. Diet and Exercise each have their place in restoring and maintaining your physical health. Dieting is how you lose weight, but exercise makes you strong and fast and durable and makes it possible for you to maintain your weight loss.

Live well,
John J. Gillies
Summer, 2009

Appendix

About the Art

Jill Krynicki did all of the illustrations. I am eternally grateful for her help. She's awesome.

Bibliography

Creating a bibliography for a book like this is difficult because I used the internet for virtually all of my research. I visited hundreds of different websites. Many of them have ceased to exist since my original visit. The sites listed below were the sites I referred to as I was building my own plan.

The Jack LaLanne Show video archives. http://www.jacklalanne.com/

Farmer Burns exercise program. http://www.sandowplus.co.uk/Competition/Burns/lessons/lesson01.htm

Kung Fu San Soo expert Harry Wong's Dynamic Strength. http://e-lacrosse.com/blogs/coaching/tag/strength/ http://en.wikipedia.org/wiki/Dynamic_Strength

Peak Conditioning (Men's Health) http://www.mothernature.com/Library/Bookshelf/Books/43/1.cfm

The Golden Age of Iron Men http://www.sandowplus.co.uk/Competition/compindex.htm#ca

The only actual books I used in the process were:
The Skinny: On Losing Weight without Being Hungry-the Ultimate Guide to Weight Loss Success by Aronne and Bowman, Published by Broadway Books, March 2009.

The Portion Teller: Smartsize Your Way to Permanent Weight Loss by Lisa R. Young. Published by Broadway Books, May 2005.
I had been experimenting with portion replacement since reading The Portion Teller: .... The Skinny: provided useful insights into changing my portion control plan.

Special mention goes to Regis Philbin, David Letterman and Rush Limbaugh. I have been following the health related stories involving Regis Philbin's coronary artery surgery, David Letterman's ongoing battle with coronary artery disease and Rush Limbaugh's struggles with his weight. I am not quite 50 years old and hope to take lessons from their ongoing health situations so that I can avoid serious problems in the future.

Yoga for Fat Guys is also published in electronic format. The electronic edition (also known as the Kindle edition) is also copyright 2009 by John J. Gillies and is also published by Sawle Register Service. ISBN: 978-0-9824750-1-0

Made in the USA
Lexington, KY
30 January 2015